MW01267777

In the Beginning

A Collection of Essays and Bible Studies on the Sanctity of Early Human Life

Foreword by Matthew C. Harrison

LCMS World Relief and Human Care

CONCORDIA PUBLISHING HOUSE • SAINT LOUIS

Written by Charles Arand, Albert Collver, Debra Grime, Arthur Just, Maggie Karner, James Lamb, Uwe Siemon-Netto, and Kevin Voss

Bible studies by James Lamb

Edited by Maggie Karner

Study concept by Robert C. Baker and Maggie Karner

This publication may be available in braille, in large print, or on cassette tape for the visually impaired. Please allow 8 to 12 weeks for delivery. Write to Lutheran Blind Mission, 7550 Watson Rd., St. Louis, MO 63119-4409; call toll-free 1-888-215-2455; or visit the Web site: www.blindmission.org.

Manufactured in the United States of America

1 2 3 4 5 6 7 8 9 10   16 15 14 13 12 11 10 09 08 07

Contents

Foreword

In 2001, the former "President's Commission on Life" (now known as the "Sanctity of Human Life Committee") found a home in LCMS World Relief and Human Care, by LCMS convention action. Amazingly, a few voices expressed consternation at the move. From our perspective, nothing could have been more appropriate. The work of LCMS World Relief and Human Care is to demonstrate mercy and compassion in the name of Christ on behalf of the Lutheran Church—Missouri Synod. Every fiber of our institutional being is about mercy toward the suffering, the needy, the least—and all this in the blessed name of Jesus. And if it is to be mercy upon the least, then let us indeed include the smallest and least.

The advance of science and technology has brought head-spinning changes and bioethics challenges. The future only promises greater complexities at a more rapid rate. This little book is a tool to help the Church to remain faithful along the way. May the very Christ who sanctified life from its beginning by taking upon Himself our flesh at every early stage and redeemed all of life—from conception to natural death and beyond—grant us wisdom and faith for this day. May He grant us courage to speak unambiguously to a world that relishes ambiguity. May He grant us courage to speak forthrightly for those who cannot speak for themselves. May He grant us love for the unloved. And may He ever have mercy upon us where we fail and bring us repentance and conviction to bear witness to life— His life—precisely where death appears to reign.

Rev. Matthew C. Harrison

Executive Director
LCMS World Relief and Human Care

Lesson 1

Creation:
Made in God's Image

Albert Collver

When the Lord God creates, He creates in His image, in His likeness. When man makes, fashions, and molds, he also does so in his image and in his likeness. Herein is the problem when we reflect on the image of God (*imago dei*). Our reflections on the image of God inevitably make the Lord God look something like us. On the surface, this may seem to be obviously true. After all, if we confess that the Lord made man in His image, it would stand to reason that a person can get an idea about God by looking at human beings, who were made in His image. Such thinking can lead us to the conclusion that we can come to know God better by knowing ourselves better. Some seek to find the image of God by looking at what is best in human beings. Others speak of the evolution of human beings as man becoming more like God. To some, the fact that human beings create, speak language, exercise dominion over the world, and have multiplied to fill the earth proves that man has the image of God. Celebrating such qualities and abilities in man tells us less about the Lord God and His image, and more about the idol we have fashioned for ourselves in our own image and likeness. We cannot discover what it means to be made in the image of God by looking to ourselves.

"In the beginning, God created the heavens and the earth" (Genesis 1:1). The Father created the heavens and the earth and all the living by speaking His Word, who is Jesus. The Holy Spirit is the Lord and giver of life. The Holy Trinity created all that exists. But the creation of man was not like the creation of all the other living things. All other living creatures came into existence when God spoke them to life. However, when it came to the creation of man, the Holy Trinity had something like a conversation that we are privileged to hear. The Scriptures only record such a conversation among the Father, Son, and Holy Spirit a few times, one of which is the creation of man. The Lord God said, "Let Us make man in Our image, after Our likeness" (Genesis 1:26). Here we see that the creation of man is different than the creation of all the other living things. The Lord even gave this "man" a name when He called him Adam.

In the creation of man, we notice the patterns that recur throughout the Scriptures. We see the Lord making something holy and setting it apart for His use and delight. When He created man, He set man apart and made him in His image and likeness, naming him Adam. The Scriptures record such special care and concern for no other creature besides man. Human beings were made in the image of God. Calamity came when man rejected that image through sin.

After the Lord God made man in His image, we are told that the serpent came to Eve. Here again we see recurring patterns. Satan tempts Eve to add or subtract from the Word of God. Specifically, he tempts her to add to what the Lord had commanded. We read that Eve adds to God's command, saying, "Do not touch the fruit." But notice that the Lord had only commanded, "Do not eat of it." Then Satan tempts her to forget a portion of the Lord's Word, namely, "Let Us make man in Our image, after Our likeness." He tempts Eve by telling her she will be "like God" (3:5). She already had been made "like God," but Satan tempted her to forget her Lord's promise. So it goes with us in our lives. We are tempted to add and to subtract from the Lord's Word. Man's desire to be like God apart from His Word caused him to lose the perfect image of God. Because man has lost the original image of God, we cannot reliably learn about that image by examining ourselves.

The true image of God can only be found in Christ Jesus, who is "the image of the invisible God" (Colossians 1:15). Jesus, "the image of God" (2 Corinthians 4:4), created man in His image (John 1:3) and now restores that image in His people. Earlier, we learned that the Scriptures occasionally record the conversations between the Father, Son, and Holy Spirit and that one of those places is the creation of man. Another place this occurs is when Jesus, nailed to the cross, cries out, "My God, My God why have You forsaken Me?" (Matthew 27:46). Jesus, the very image of God, is forsaken by His Father. Here, Jesus is forsaken because in His passion He became just like us who have lost the image of God. We see Him take our lost and fallen image upon Himself. Now He restores the lost image of God by setting us apart and putting His name upon us in the waters of Holy Baptism. In the Sacrament of Holy Baptism, the Christian is given the image of Christ—the image of the crucified Christ in this life, and the image of the resurrected Christ in the life to come (Romans 6).

This image of God has profound implications for how we treat our neighbor. Perhaps first and foremost is the recognition that Christ died for our neighbor, without regard to any merit or worthiness in him. In your neighbor is a person that Christ desires to restore and to remake in the image of God.

In today's scientifically complex society, we can also see how we often strive to create in our own image. Rather than receiving our neighbor as a gift, we seek to remake (or even unmake) him according to our desired image of the human being. If our neighbor's existence, disabilities, size, or problems offend our image of the human being, we can easily dismiss him and treat him as less than human or regard ourselves as better than him.

The basis for how we treat our neighbor is twofold. The Law of God commands us not to hurt or harm our neighbor in his body but to help and befriend him in every bodily need. This command is given to all human beings and is enforced by threat of punishment and fear. Yet the Christian who is remade in the image of Christ has the motivation of Christ's underserved love and mercy. Just as Christ loved us and redeemed us, even though we had no merit or worthiness in us, we, too, love our neighbor and show mercy to others. Christ seeks the unlovable; He sought unlovable us and now we—who have been set apart and named in Holy Baptism—show mercy to those the world considers unlovable, unwanted, inconvenient, and unworthy of life. Because Christ has recreated us in His image, we see in our neighbor a person whom Jesus also wants to redeem and transform into His image—a person whom only Jesus can restore to the image of God.

The Value of Life and the Image of God

James Lamb

Does human life have intrinsic value? If so, when does that value begin? Answering these two questions is critical in dealing with a variety of issues related to modern technologies and human life at its very beginnings. Anyone can postulate that human life has intrinsic value from the very beginning. But only Christians can articulate "why"—in a way no one else can. Christians can go beyond intrinsic value and talk of *God-given* intrinsic value. The answer to the question, "What has God done that gives value to human life from the very beginning?" is the focus of this series of studies.

Image Given

1. Read Genesis 1:26–27. From the very beginning, God's action elevates human life above all other life. What particular things in these verses testify to this?

2. Read Psalm 8. This psalm praises the majestic name of God (vv. 1, 9). The reason for this praise is the "work of Your fingers," God's creation (v. 3). The creation of human life is included as part of this work. Where do you find Genesis 1:26–27 reflected in this psalm?

3. Read Genesis 2:7 and 2:22. Note the action words associated with the creation of Adam and Eve in God's image. God "formed" Adam and "breathed" into him. He "made" (literally "built") Eve. How do these words help enhance the value given to the first humans?

4. Read Genesis 9:6 and James 3:9. In the next section, we will study how the original image of God was lost. Nevertheless, even after the fall, this original, lofty position of being the "work of [God's] fingers" still gives value. How would Grandma's handmade quilt that is proudly displayed although old and tattered relate to this?

Image Lost

5. Read Genesis 3:1–7. The "glory and honor" of this original image, however, is short-lived. Evil enters God's perfect world and confronts His perfect people. What is the essence of Satan's temptation (v. 5)?

6. Of course, Adam and Eve already were like God. But Satan cleverly adds, "knowing good and evil." It's as if Satan is saying, "Why should God have a monopoly on what is right and wrong? Why can't you get in on that?" Satan convinces Adam and Eve, who were perfect and who had a perfect knowledge of God, that things could actually be *better*! But what did this "new

knowledge" lead to? Consider Genesis 2:17; Genesis 3:7, 10; Romans 8:7–8; and Genesis 5:3.

The Image of Man

7. Read Genesis 6:5. How do things progress for those born in the image and likeness of Adam?

8. How is God treated? (See Romans 1:23.)

Not only does our fallen nature want to remake God into some other image, but, as Dr. Collver states in his essay, "If our neighbor's existence, disabilities, size, or problems offend our image of the human being, we can easily dismiss him and treat him as less than human or regard ourselves as better than him." Discuss this in relation to James 1:27–2:4.

Seeking the Lost

9. Read Genesis 3:9. Adam and Eve lost the image of God and it was no longer part of their being to be passed along to their offspring. The pure knowledge of God and their holiness was lost. Human beings began a long, disturbing road of judging God and their neighbor in terms of their own likeness and image. That God still loves and values the human lives He created, however, is seen in His action here. What is God doing in this verse that He did not have to do?

Discuss Luke 19:10 and John 15:1–24 in relation to this.

Promising the Lost

10. Read Genesis 3:15. God reveals in this promise the means He would use for humankind's restoration. Relate the word *offspring* to Galatians 4:4 and Luke 1:29–33.

11. God revealed in this promise the price He would pay for this restoration. Relate the words *bruise His heel* to Isaiah 53:3–5 and Matthew 27:45–46.

Conclusion

This promise is for all humanity. Discuss the implications regarding the value of every human life and how we treat our neighbor. Dr. Collver puts it this way: "In your neighbor is a person that Christ desires to restore and remake in the image of God." This restoration through justification is the topic of Lesson 2.

Lesson 2

Justification: Life through His Word

Charles P. Arand

We find ourselves in hundreds of small "courtrooms" every day of our lives. In them, we constantly encounter accusations such as What were you thinking? or Why did you do that? These questions require that we justify or vindicate ourselves to other people, and perhaps also to ourselves. Statements like *You are hired/You are fired* and *I love you/I hate you* deeply affect us. In the twenty-first century, we now find ourselves in a position of not only having to justify ourselves in the eyes of others, but having to justify the existence of those who are too helpless to defend themselves—those at the beginning of life as well as those suffering from debilitating diseases at the end of life. As important as human judgments are, in the end, it is God who has the final word. Ultimately, it is His judgment that determines the reality of our existence and defines our worth. What He says about us makes what others say about us merely provisional. What He says about us alone frees us from our own self-evaluation. In brief, His life-giving and life-justifying Word bestows upon us an inestimable value and worth as God's human creatures.

Luther knew what it was like to live under the judging eye of God. He was reminded of that fact every time he entered the city church in Wittenberg. On a stone relief above the entrance to the cemetery by the church, Luther saw an angry Christ seated on the rainbow as judge of the world. He believed that winning a favorable judgment from God was anything but certain. A German catechist on the eve of the Reformation expressed the uncertainty of the age, "There are three things I know to be true that frequently make my heart heavy. The first troubles my spirit, because I will have to die. The second troubles my heart more, because I do not know when. The third troubles me above all. I do not know where I will go."[1] The uncertainty drove Luther to despair, because he realized that he could not face Christ as his judge and survive no matter how hard he tried to live a holy life with the assistance of God's grace and the Church's guidance.

And yet, Luther arrived at the point where he could joyfully pray, "Come, dear last day." This occurred when he realized that the Gospel does not reveal a righteousness demanded from us by God, but a righteousness that God bestows upon us (Romans 1:17). Luther came to see that love, not wrath, constituted the core of God's being. The reason for this is that God gave His Son to take our sins upon Himself as if they were His own. Luther describes this in vivid language, "Now He is not the Son of God, born of the Virgin. But He is a sinner, who has and bears the sin of Paul, the former blasphemer, persecutor, and assaulter; of Peter, who denied Christ; of David, who was an adulterer and a murderer, and who caused the Gentiles to blaspheme the name of the Lord" (LW 26:277).[2] In the death of Christ, "God has rendered his verdict upon sin; it is evil, and it must be destroyed."[3] By raising Christ from the dead, God made Him our righteousness (Romans 4:25; LW 26:21–22).

On account of Christ's death and resurrection, God announced His vindication of the world through the promise of the Gospel. In it, God unconditionally guarantees that He will receive us into the new age as His children. Most importantly, the Gospel is not a promise that will be fulfilled only in the future; it is a creative Word that takes immediate effect now—in the present time. It announces that we have gone through God's judgment ahead of time. God's Word does what it says. God's justifying Word does not define the status of the believer "as if" she was righteous. Instead, when God declares a person to be righteous, that person is really righteous. He clothes a person with the righteousness of Christ. As Luther expressed it, "above this life I have another righteousness, another life, which is

---

[1] Denis Janz, *Three Reformation Catechisms: Catholic, Anabaptist, Lutheran* (New York: Mellen, 1982), 127.

[2] "Galatians Lectures," 1531–1535, *Luther's Works* (Saint Louis/Philadelphia: Concordia/Fortress, 1958–1986) [henceforth LW]

[3] Robert Kolb, "Luther's Theology of the Cross," *Lutheran Quarterly*, 16 (2002): 454.

Christ."[4] This Word recreates us as people who live in complete dependence upon Him. Jesus called this gift of identity from God "new birth" or "birth from above" (John 3:3). These images stress that in our relationship with God we are passive. We simply trust Him and rely upon His Word of validation.

The Word that freely justifies us is the same Word that first gave us physical life. Luther liked to say that God has His own grammar when He speaks. His words are not like our words—words that are spoken into thin air. Instead, God's words make things happen. Commenting on Psalm 2, Luther states, "And when He speaks, the mountains tremble, kingdoms are scattered, then indeed the whole earth is moved" (LW 12:32–33). God's Word says what it does and does what it says. Indeed, by His Word God "calls into existence the things that do not exist" (Romans 4:17). When He said, "let there be," He brought all things into existence (Genesis 1:2, 6, 9, 11, 14, 20, 24, 26). "When [God] says 'Sun, shine,' the sun is there at once and shines" (LW 1:21–22). Accordingly, the words of God are not full of hot air, but are "things very great and wonderful, which we see with our eyes and feel with our hands" (LW 12:32). This means that human life is a life that depends on God and God's Word.

God's Word did not bring about all things only at the initial moment of creation, but embraced the entire creation that followed. "For when God once said (Genesis 1:28): 'Be fruitful,' that Word is effective to this day and preserves nature in a miraculous way" (LW 4:4). There is a sense for Luther that God already created those of us who live in the twenty-first century when His Word created the entire world (Genesis 1–2). Speaking of himself, Luther reflected:

> In God's sight I was begotten and multiplied immediately when the world began, because this Word, "and God said: 'Let Us make man,'" created me too. Whatever God wanted to create, that He created then when He spoke. Not everything has come into view at once. Similarly, an arrow or a ball which is shot from a cannon (for it has greater speed) is sent to its target in a single moment, as it were, and nevertheless it is shot through a definite space; so God, through His

---

[4] LW [*Luther's Works*] 26:9.

Word, extends His activity from the beginning of the world to its end. (LW 1:76)

For this reason, Luther describes God's Word as being "without end" (LW 1:75) and remaining effective to this day. For Luther, God's creative Word runs through the past, present, and future and binds them together (LW 1:76). In God's eyes, all things are present to Him at the same time.

Today, God's action is usually perceived only through the mediation of creatures. They become God's "masks"—instruments of His Word, by which He creates us. And so our existence, as human creatures, was given to us by God through our parents. They conceived us, and our mothers gave us birth, without any active participation on our part. We were completely passive even though we came from our mother's womb kicking and crying. In the Small Catechism, Luther draws his characteristic language for justification into the article on creation when he elegantly confesses, "God has created me . . . out of His pure, fatherly, and divine goodness and mercy, without any merit or worthiness on my part." That is how it has been since the very beginning. "Adam and Eve were not given a probationary period in which to demonstrate that they were worthy of their humanity. It could not be earned. It was a gift. . . . It must be passively received.[5] Another way of saying this is that, when God created heaven and earth out of nothing, God established His relationship with us. A relationship of His unconstrained giving to our absolute receiving. As with justification, our very creation is dependent on God's gracious self-giving and creating within the world.

The Word justifies our human existence and defines our human worth. As the Word brought about the creation of Adam and Eve, the Word makes the sinner righteous by giving us the gifts of Christ. Made in the image of God, human beings were created as unique creatures who grasped and reflected God's goodness by living in complete confidence of and total reliance upon God. With His Word, God has placed His divine stamp of approval upon His human creatures. "The unassailable worth of each individual applies unconditionally to all human persons.

---

[5] Kolb, "Luther's Theology of the Cross," 412.

This worth is unmerited, and therefore cannot be lost. It is promised and God's promise cannot be rescinded; it is, as it were, an indelible character."[6]

[6] Johannes Schwanke, "Luther on Creation," *Harvesting Martin Luther's Reflections on Theology, Ethics, and the Church*, ed. Timothy J. Wengert (Grand Rapids: Eerdmans, 2004), 97.

The Value of Life and the Restored Image of God

James Lamb

As we saw in Lesson 1, God loved what He made in His image so much that when the image was lost He promised to send a Savior who would restore it. All of Scripture, from Genesis through Revelation, reveals what God did through His Word made flesh, Jesus Christ, to justify sinners and purchase for them a righteousness they did not deserve and could never earn. His creative Word becomes a re-creative Word in Jesus. This justification by grace through faith becomes the thread running through all of Scripture. What God did in Christ to restore lost humanity gives value to all humanity. As Dr. Arand states in his essay, "In brief, His life-giving and life-justifying Word bestows upon us an inestimable value and worth as God's human creatures" (p. 12). This study looks at what is involved in restoring the image of God.

Image Reversal

Read Romans 8:3. Because there was a "first Adam," God chose to send a "last Adam." (See 1 Corinthians 15:21–22, 45.)

12. How inclusive is the death that the first Adam brought?

13. How inclusive is the life that the last Adam brought?

To restore the likeness and image of God in fallen humankind, Jesus took upon Himself human nature. (See also Philippians 2:6–7 and Hebrews 2:14–15.)

Reversal Reasons

14. What reasons for this image reversal are given in the following verses: 2 Corinthians 5:21; Galatians 3:10–13; and Matthew 27:46?

Reversal's Scope

Review the universal love of God in the following passages: John 3:16; 1 Timothy 2:1–6; and 1 Peter 3:18.

This image reversal took place for all humanity. Every human being is a human being for whom Jesus lived, died, and rose again. This gives value to every human being from the very beginning of their humanity. This makes every human being our neighbor whom we are to love as ourselves.

Image Renewal

15. Read Romans 3:19–26. Of course, the image reversal does not stop with Jesus taking our image—He gives us His! This happens by His grace through faith. According to these verses, when God looks at the believer, whose image does He see?

Renewal of Knowledge

16. Read Colossians 3:9–10. The perfect knowledge of God given to Adam and Eve is being renewed in the believer. Our first parents had this knowledge "built in." How do we receive it (2 Corinthians 4:6; Romans 3:22)?

Renewal of Holiness

17. Read Ephesians 4:24. The perfect holiness in which Adam and Eve were created to be like God is part of our "new self, created after the likeness of God." How do we "put on" this new self (1 Peter 2:1–3; Romans 6:4; 1 Corinthians 11:23–26)?

Renewal Is a Process

18. Read 2 Corinthians 3:18. A pastor once preached a sermon with the theme "Now—Not Yet." Right now we are being renewed into the image of God through Christ, but that image is not yet fully restored. Contrast the "Now—Not Yet" of Paul by looking at Galatians 2:20 and then Romans 7:18–20.

Image Restored

19. Read 2 Corinthians 4:16–18 and Revelation 21:1–4. Because of the work of Christ, we can be assured that, as another pastor used to share with his homebound members, "The best is yet to come." Discuss this "best" and the hope it gives.

Conclusion

The Bible begins and ends with human beings bearing the image of God and living in perfection. What happens in between is what God did in Jesus Christ to restore at the end what was lost in the beginning. What happens in between is a testament to the immeasurable value God gives to human life from the very beginning.

Lesson 3

Incarnation: Being Like Us in Every Way

Arthur Just

By creating us in His image, God shows us that our true humanity is to be like Him—perfect and without sin. But when everything went wrong in the garden, what was so good became polluted with the virus of sin. In order to make right what had gone wrong, the One who created us in His image must enter our creation and be like us in every way, but without sin. Jesus, the Son of God, our Creator, must become flesh to show us what our true humanity looks like in His perfect, sinless being.

When the angel Gabriel greeted the Virgin Mary saying, "Rejoice, O favored one, the Lord is with you" (Luke 1:28), Mary knew that she was in the presence of a great mystery. She knew this greeting was reserved by the Old Testament prophets only for the Daughter of Zion. How could she be addressed by an angel sent from God, a humble, teenage virgin from Nazareth of Galilee? No wonder she was troubled at this word and pondered what sort of greeting this might be.

After announcing to her that she would bear a son, the angel instructed her as to the character of her child. Mary was no fool. Any child called Jesus, the Savior from sins—any child called Great, Son of the Most High, eternal King over the house of Jacob—could be none other than the promised Messiah, the Christ. Could it be? Could she, Mary, be the final link in the chain of Old Testament genealogies, Israel reduced to one, the mother of the Messiah? Could she, Mary, a humble, teenage virgin from Nazareth, be the God-bearer?

Mary was no fool. She asked the biological question. "How will this be, since I am a virgin?" (Luke 1:34). The angel answered by speaking into her ear and bringing about the greatest mystery of all—the incarnation of Jesus Christ our Savior: "The Holy Spirit will come upon you, and the power of the Most High will overshadow you" (Luke 1:35). This same Spirit hovered over the waters and brought forth creation (Genesis 1:2), over Israel as the presence of God in the pillar of cloud (the *shekinah*) during the exodus (Exodus 13; 14; 33), over the ark of the covenant (Exodus 40), at Sinai (Exodus 19), over Jesus at His Baptism (Luke 3), and in the cloud at His transfiguration (Luke 9). This same Spirit would also be promised to the disciples by Jesus just before His ascension, when they will be "clothed with power from on high" (Luke 24:49). As the angel spoke the Word to Mary, the Holy Spirit came upon her and overshadowed her, and she conceived Jesus as holy, the Son of God. From the moment of His conception, Jesus was both God and man.

For Martin Luther, the Word the angel spoke was the moment of conception. He answers the biological question for Mary and for us. She conceived through her ear, through the very Word of God, that same Word of God that the Holy Spirit uses to conceive Christ in us. "So faith comes from hearing, and hearing through the word of Christ" (Romans 10:17).

The mystery deepens. The power of the Most High that overshadowed Mary is the same word used to describe the pillar of cloud that overshadowed the tabernacle, signaling the presence and glory of Yahweh. Mary was not only the new Israel, she was now the new temple—not because of who she was, but because of what she bore in her womb. And the angel confirmed it: "The child to be born will be called holy—the Son of God" (Luke 1:35). Mary's womb was now the Holy of Holies, for God dwelled there in the flesh.

The Annunciation to the Virgin Mary teaches us about the virgin birth—Jesus as the Son of God, the work of the Holy Spirit in Jesus' conception. And because we are in Him and He is in us, the sanctity of our own human life begins at the moment of conception. The Nicene Creed captures all this teaching in a single phrase: Jesus "was incarnate by the Holy Spirit of the Virgin Mary and was made man." As "Son of God" and "holy," Jesus is set apart by God to cleanse Israel—and all of us—from our sins and to inherit for us the kingdom promised by the Father. Unlike Jesus, the words of David apply to us: "Behold, I was brought forth in iniquity, and in sin did my mother conceive me" (Psalm 51:5). Our perfect humanity has been infected with sin from the very beginning, from the moment of our conception. So we needed our Creator to return with His perfect humanity, who was brought forth by the Holy Spirit, conceived in His mother's womb but without sin, by the power of the Most High. Jesus was required to go from conception to death, just like us.

Upon hearing the news of Jesus' conception in her womb, Mary traveled into the hill country of Judea to visit her cousin Elizabeth, who was ready to give birth to John the Baptist. Mary's journey was paralleled by the movement of the ark of the covenant to the same locale on its way to Jerusalem. As a temporary and portable vessel housing the immanent presence of the true God in her womb, for a time Mary appears to fulfill the purpose of the ark of the covenant. The child in Mary's womb "is appointed for the fall and rising of many in Israel, and for a sign that is opposed" (Luke 2:34). Conceived by the Holy Spirit, and occupying a holy womb, Jesus is the mercy seat where blood will be poured out to cleanse all those conceived in sin and brought forth in iniquity.

When Mary entered Elizabeth's house, everything that happened was a response to the presence of God in the flesh—the Baby inside Mary. The presence of the Lord causes John the Baptist to leap in the womb of Elizabeth, a sign already that Jesus the Creator affects the creation by His presence. The "fleshly" presence of the Messiah, the agent of all creation, causes great things to take place within God's creation. Here we see the new creation beginning, and a baby, still in the womb, hails the new creation's inception. In John's leap, the miracles of Jesus are foreshadowed. For this Jesus caused all creation to leap at His presence: "the blind receive their sight, the lame walk, lepers are cleansed, and the deaf hear, the dead are raised up, the poor have good news preached to them" (Luke 7:22). Even from the womb, John prophecies:

> Not yet born, already John prophesies and, while still in the enclosure of his mother's womb, confesses the coming of Christ with movements of joy—since he could not do so with his voice. As Elizabeth says to holy Mary: "As soon as you greeted me, the child in

my womb exulted for joy."[7] John exults, then, before he is born. Before his eyes can see what the world looks like, he can recognize the Lord of the world with his spirit. In this regard, I think that the prophetic phrase is appropriate: "Before I formed you in the womb I knew you, and before you came forth from the womb I sanctified you."[8] Thus we ought not to marvel that, after Herod put him in prison, he continued to announce Christ to his disciples from his confinement, when even confined in the womb he preached the same Lord by his movements.[9]

Elizabeth was so overcome by the presence of Mary and the child in her womb that she exclaimed to Mary: "Blessed are you among women, and blessed is the fruit of your womb!" (Luke 1:42). Mary, daughter of Eve and Sarah and "Zion," is truly "blessed." She is unique because the "fruit" of her "womb" is the God and Savior of the entire human race (cf. Titus 2:13). She is *theotokos*—the "mother of God."[10] Two women, one very young and one very old, are chosen by God for His miraculous purpose of bearing and nurturing the two most important figures in salvation history.

These two figures, conceived by the power of the Holy Spirit, show us that human life begins at conception. Even in the womb, Jesus, the Creator and Redeemer of all things, is working His new creation. And John, the forerunner and final Old Testament prophet, responds to His Lord's presence by leaping in the womb. In utero, John and Jesus declare the truth that life begins at conception and is to be sanctified by all.

---

[7] Luke 1:44.
[8] Jeremiah 1:5.
[9] Maximus of Turin, Sermon 5.4, On the Birthday of John the Baptist, ACW 50:24.
[10] (FC Ep VIII 12; FC SD VIII 24).

The Incarnation and the Value of Life

James Lamb

When does human life begin? Embryology textbooks used in medical schools make the answer clear. "Zygote: This cell results from the union of an oocyte and a sperm. A zygote is the beginning of a new human being (i.e., an embryo)."[11]

There is no better place in Scripture to affirm this scientific fact than the incarnation of Jesus. We will look to Scripture for the what, who, how, and why of the incarnation, and then see how these attest to the value of all human life from the moment of conception.

What Is the Incarnation?

Read John 1:14; Hebrews 2:14; and 1 Timothy 3:16 and answer the questions.

20. Who was the Word? Who shared our humanity? Who appeared in the flesh?

The answer, of course, is the Sunday School answer—Jesus! But there is something much more profound here. Read Philippians 2:5–8. The incarnation is much more than something becoming flesh or someone becoming flesh. The incarnation is God becoming flesh!

---

[11] Keith L. Moore and T.V.N. Persaud, *The Developing Human* (Philadelphia: W.B. Saunders Company, 1998), 2.

Who Was Involved?

God did not just suddenly "take over" someone's body like we see in alien movies. God "became" our flesh! For that, He needed to begin where humanity begins. He needed human flesh, a fallopian tube, and a womb!

21. Read Luke 1:26–28. What is significant about the following:

a. Nazareth—(See Matthew 2:23 and John 1:45)

b. Virgin—(See Isaiah 7:13–14)

c. Joseph, a descendant of David—(See 1 Samuel 7:5, 11, 16 and Luke 1:32)

d. "Rejoice, O favored one, the Lord is with you."—(See Dr. Just's essay, p. 20, paragraph two.)

22. Read Luke 1:29–33. We often read verse 31 as one event at Christmas. But how many events are described? How long between them? What do we celebrate on March 25?

23. Relate the first event to Genesis 3:15. What is significant about the names "Jesus" and "Son of the Most High"? (See Dr. Just's essay and Matthew 1:21.)

24. Why is it appropriate to call Mary the "mother of God"?

How Did It Happen?

25. Read Luke 1:34–38. Mary asks a logical and biological question. The ordinary process of sperm uniting with egg will not be operative here. What *extra*-ordinary process will be used instead (v. 35)?

Herein lays the miracle of the incarnation! The miracle of Christmas is that God would be born in such humble conditions. Wondrous signs accompany His birth—angel choirs in fields and a special star overhead. But the birth itself, from a biological point of view, was just like any other birth. The miracle of God becoming man had happened nine months earlier!

26. Test your understanding! In the Holy Land, an inscription on a wall reads, "Here the Word became flesh." Can you guess the town where this inscription is found?[12]

---

[12] Answer: Nazareth.

That Mary was pregnant with God by the power of the Holy Spirit from the moment of conception was verified when she went to visit Elizabeth.

27. Read Luke 1:39–45. What is baby John's reaction to Mary's greeting (v. 41)?

28. What very human emotion does John exhibit (v. 44)?

29. It would probably take Mary six to seven days to travel to Elizabeth's house. Do a little "biology research." How big was Jesus? Where was Jesus?[13]

30. How does Elizabeth refer to Mary (v. 43)?

31. In Luke 1, note all the places where "Lord" is used. To whom does it always refer?

Why Did It Happen?

Jesus became flesh at the moment of conception because of a problem with our conception (see Psalm 51:5).

---

[13] Answers: Around 110 cells; most likely in Mary's fallopian tube or just recently having reached her uterus.

If we are sinful from the moment of conception, we are human and in need of a Savior from the moment of conception.

32. Read Hebrews 2:14, concentrating this time on the last half of the verse. What did it take to "destroy the one who has the power of death"?

What Are the Implications of the Incarnation of Jesus to Human Beginnings?

Discuss the following. Every time you recite the words of the Apostles' Creed, "conceived by the Holy Spirit," or the Nicene Creed, "was incarnate by the Holy Spirit of the Virgin Mary and was made man," you are attesting to Jesus' divinity at the moment of conception, and also to our humanity at the moment of conception.

33. Do Jesus' conception in Mary's fallopian tube and the events that took place at Elizabeth's house when Jesus was probably still traveling in that fallopian tube speak to what is called today "pre-implantation human life"?

34. Should human embryos in a petri dish or frozen in a fertility clinic be afforded the same dignity as those in fallopian tubes or wombs? (The key to the answer is in the word *human*.)

Conclusion

The embryology textbooks are clear. Based on the incarnation, how does Scripture answer the question, When does human life begin? This is the focus of our next lesson.

Lesson 4

Conception:
A Medical Analysis
of Early Life

Debra Grime

"What are these balls called again?" my curious son asked during bath time. "Testicles," I replied, trying to encourage proper medical terminology. "Oh, yeah. That's where my seeds are made." "Sperm," I corrected. "Yeah, yeah. Hey, exactly how many seeds do I have?" "Oh, I don't know," I replied, deciding he was too young to explain that spermatogenesis doesn't occur until adolescence. "Well God knows!" he shouted. "He knows everything. My teacher showed us in the Bible that God knows the number of hairs on my head. So if He has counted every hair, I'm sure He has counted all my seeds. He knows exactly how many seeds I have. That means He knows how many babies I'm going to have. I bet I'm going to have millions!" Although most of us don't think about God bothering to count our eggs and sperm, my boy was right. God does know everything about us. Down to the last egg.

Let's look at how these special cells are formed. Controlled by hormones, the testicles in men and the ovaries in women develop *gametes*, a generic term for *eggs* and *sperm*. These two processes are called *spermatogenesis* and *oogenesis*.

Each sperm or egg contains 23 chromosomes, half of what you need to start human life. Every cell in our bodies contains 46 chromosomes except for the gametes. Each egg has 23 X chromosomes. The egg can only contribute the sex chromosome X. In contrast, sperm can either be 23 X or 23 Y. If a 23 X sperm is combined with a 23 X egg, a 46 XX fertilized egg will form and the child will be a girl. If a 23 Y sperm is combined with a 23 X egg, a 46 XY fertilized egg will form and the child will be a boy.

"Why don't I look like my brother?" my adopted boys questioned. "Well, you each were born to different women." "Oh yeah. So I have half of my biological mother and half of my biological father and he has half of his biological mother and half of his biological father." "Right," I said, thinking about how many times I've had to explain this. Thankfully, they were finally putting the pieces together, as difficult as that can be emotionally for them. "But Mom, how come my friends, who aren't adopted and who come from the same mom and dad, don't look exactly like their brothers?" (Medical school doesn't prepare you for parenting!) "Remember how women have eggs and men have sperm?" I began. "Well, as they are formed, a process called crossing over occurs. Part of the chromosomes come apart and rejoin to make a new combination. The genetic material, which determines what you look like and many other traits, is shuffled around. This gives each sperm and egg a unique and special chromosomal combination. It means that some of the children's traits may be the same or similar to a parent, but others will be different." Like shuffling a deck of cards, each hand will be different, yet some of the cards could be the same. Unlike a deck of cards where no new cards are added, with marriage, new genetic material or DNA in the chromosomes is introduced, allowing for even more variations. In crossing over, I see God's unlimited potential for creativity. There is only one me, yet I am physically connected to my family through mutual DNA . . . and to the human race by our common human genome.

In medical school, we frequently received notices inquiring if we would sell our eggs or sperm to infertility clinics. They needed gametes and most of us needed money. God isn't the only one counting sperm and valuing their unique and special potential. I asked a fellow student if he had ever considered making a "contribution." "I get more as a gigolo," he teased. Then he got serious and said, "Never would do it. I want to know where my sperm is going. I can't imagine not knowing when, where, and with whom my 'deposit' was being made. Too many questions would haunt me. Was it successful? Do I have children? Even if I'm not legally responsible for them, those children would be a part of me." He didn't want to be disconnected from a part of himself. Connections and interconnections are part of being human.

Microscopically, our first connection was at conception. We wouldn't be here if somebody's egg and somebody's sperm hadn't united. Once that one in a million sperm, hand-chosen by God, penetrates into a special egg, there is no going back. There is no natural unhooking. It's "until death do thee part." The sperm can't say to the egg, "This was nice but I really don't want to be committed." In conception, a set of 23 unique chromosomes makes a permanent connection with another unique set of 23 chromosomes to form a new 46-chromosome cell called a *fertilized egg*, a *zygote*, or an *embryo*. This is day 1 of human life.

Human life has its beginning with this 46-chromosome zygote. It has started its own unique timeline. In natural conception, this occurs in the fallopian tube of the mother's uterus. As this new life travels along the fallopian tube, it is busy dividing and growing. First it divides into 2 cells, then 4, then 8, and then into 16 cells in the form of a ball called a *morula*. By day 5, the morula has changed, hollowing out to form a fluid-filled cavity. It is now called a *blastocyst*. By day 6, the blastocyst has entered the uterine cavity and comes to rest upon the prepared uterine wall. Implantation begins and is completed around day 14. Cells begin to migrate and differentiate into precursors of the tissue from which organs will develop. By day 22, the heart starts to beat. Spinal column, head, arms, legs, eyes, ears, and nose all begin to develop. By week 7, we frequently measure the developing baby by ultrasound machines to date the pregnancy. The baby continues to maturate at a predictable rate. From day 1 at fertilization, it's on a continuum of cell division, maturation, and change. From the fallopian tube; to the womb; to the delivery table and mother's arms, to the crib, to the preschool, elementary, and high school; to college and later to a career; followed by the midlife crisis; to the nursing home; and finally the tomb— an individual, personal timeline forms. As we ponder our life's length and capacity, we remember that God planned our timelines. "Your eyes saw my unformed substance; in Your book were written, every one of them, the days that were formed for me, when as yet there were none of them" (Psalm 139:16).

It is interesting that conception microscopically mirrors marriage. The male sperm leaves his testicular home and unites with the female egg and they become one new cell, a zygote. The two become one—literally! What a profound mystery! As God unites man and wife, so He brings together sperm and egg. "Your hands have made me and fashioned me," writes the psalmist (Psalm 119:73). What God has joined together, dare we separate?

However, conception, the microscopic union once only seen by God, can now be seen and manipulated by scientists and medical specialists. Some common infertility treatments are *in vitro fertilization* (IVF), *gamete intrafallopian transfer* (GIFT), *zygote intrafallopian transfer* (ZIFT), and *intracytoplasmic sperm injection* (ICSI). Briefly, let's look at their definitions.

IVF: Sperm and eggs are collected and brought together in a special medium in a petri dish. Sperm spontaneously fertilize the eggs, forming zygotes. The zygotes are allowed to divide and are then placed into the uterus, where it is hoped they will implant and continue to grow.

GIFT: Gametes, both eggs and sperm, are collected and placed together into a catheter. They are both placed into the fallopian tube, where fertilization occurs.

ZIFT: Eggs are fertilized in vitro and some of the resulting fertilized eggs are inserted into a fallopian tube.

ICSI: Sperm and eggs are collected. Using microsurgical techniques, a single sperm is injected into an egg. The fertilized egg is allowed to grow and is placed into the uterus.

Some ethical issues that are faced when using infertility technology include the issue of donor gametes (sperm and/or eggs used from people other than husband and wife); selling gametes or the use of "leftover" embryos from IVF for embryonic stem cell research; embryo freezing and embryo losses from thawing; experimentation with embryos; and embryo testing for genetic abnormalities.

The desire for children is natural and God-given. In Genesis 1:28, we read, "And God blessed them. And God said to them, 'Be fruitful and multiply and fill the earth.'" After sin entered the world, creation had disease and malformations. Couples were sometimes unable to have children. As we look at infertility, we see not only the extreme personal sadness of not being able to have a child, but also the extreme distance that sin created between us and God. God desires a relationship and direct connections with us. Sin disrupts this connection and our connections with family and others. Christ had to come to be our mediator, to reconnect us to God. That doesn't mean that all of creation is perfect again. But it does mean that through Baptism we belong to God's family, carrying the name of the Father, Son, and Holy Spirit. We can look at these issues and be reminded that God is the Creator of heaven and earth . . . that *He* "has given me my body and soul, eyes, ears and all my members, my reason and all my senses."

The Work of His Hands and the Value of Life

James Lamb

The Work of His Hands—Adam and Eve

In Lesson 1, we looked briefly at Genesis 2 and God's "hands-on" creation of Adam and Eve. Let's review and expand on that.

35. Read Genesis 2:7 and 2:22. What "hands-on" picture do you get of the creation of Adam?

36. What other intimate detail makes the giving of life special?

37. What "hands-on" picture do you get of the creation of Eve? (Remember, "made" literally means "built.")

38. What does Genesis 1:28 imply about how human life will come into existence from now on?

39. Discuss the importance of the *context* for this biological procreative process. (See Genesis 2:24.)

The Work of His Hands—All Human Life

The biology God established is much more than what is commonly referred to as *reproduction*. The word *reproduction* reminds us of a factory assembly line. We should remember that humans are more than products. We are individual creations! As described in the essay, God uses the wonderful intricacies of this biology to continue His "hands-on" work in *procreation* or "creating forth."

A brief study of Psalm 139 will help connect the biological fact that human life begins at conception with the scriptural truth that God involves Himself in the formation of human life from the very beginning.

"Big Brother"?

At first, Psalm 139 may seem a little frightening, like "Big Brother" knowing and watching everything you do.

40. Read Psalm 139:1–6. Discuss the things God knows about you. What could be disconcerting about this?

41. Read Psalm 139:7–12. What do these verses say about God's presence?

42. It is nice to think about our ever-present God. On the other hand, what might be scary about God always being around?

Creator God!

Read Psalm 139:13. It's not frightening after all! God does not watch as a menacing "Big Brother." He watches as your loving Creator. God knows you because He was intimately involved in your formation. He does not watch over you trying to catch you in some mistake. He watches over you because He made you and loves you.

The phrase translated "inward parts" (ESV) or "inmost being" (NIV) or "possessed my reins" (KJV) literally comes out something like "you made (or possessed) my kidneys"! The kidneys were the last organs removed in sacrificial disemboweling, the "inward parts." This idiom speaks to that which is "you" at your very essence.

43. Keeping in mind the biology of Dr. Grime's essay, when did "you" become a unique individual?

44. The psalm progresses: "You knitted me together in my mother's womb." Literally translated, this means, "You wove a covering for me." Again, remembering the biology, what begins to develop after "you" implant in the uterus and cells begin to "migrate and differentiate"?

45. So God creates you at the moment of conception and then weaves a covering for you: your body! Discuss this: What happens to you if the cells God uses to weave your covering are removed for research purposes?

46. Read Psalm 139:14. We might get confused trying to

understand the complexity of the biology involved in all this. But David gives us a good alternative. What does he do?

47. How do these words give value to human life?

48. Read Psalm 139:15–16. David returns to God's intimate knowledge of us. What is the "secret" place?

49. This parallels "depths of the earth," another Hebrew idiom for the dark, damp, secret place of the womb from which life comes.
According to verse 16, when did God know you as you?

50. How does this verse reveal the problems with the statement, "Well, an embryo doesn't look like a human being!"?

51. God knew you from your very beginning. What did He also know *about* you?

52. So, when a human embryo is destroyed, what else is lost?

53. Read Psalm 139:17–18. Why does God's presence bring comfort and not fear? Discuss this in relation to John 16:7–11.

54. Read Psalm 139:19–22. It seems like these verses are from another psalm! But David's anger is kindled against those who would rise up against God. Rising up against the work of His hands is rising up against Him. When we consider the destruction of human embryos in the name of "good" and the killing of the unborn in the name of "choice," is there a place for such righteous anger?

55. Read Psalm 139:23–24. David prays in the final verses for what he acknowledged in the first verse—that God would search his heart and thoughts. We can and should be angry, but our anger should not lead us to sin. Anger is not the basis for sharing the truth of God's Word. What is (Ephesians 4:15)?

56. Where does such love come from (1 John 4:9–11)?

Conclusion

Conclude by discussing the *positive* messages from Psalm 139 that we can use to defend and protect "the work of His hands" from the very beginning.

Lesson 5

Science:
The Truth and Hype
about Stem Cells

Kevin Voss

As I am writing this essay, *embryonic stem cell research* (ESCR) is in the news again. As I travel the country speaking on this topic, it is apparent to me that many Christians are confused by this issue and wondering what the controversy is all about. They know that the religious leaders of many conservative Christian denominations are opposed to ESCR, but they don't really know why. In today's post-modern world, Christians have been thrust into a sometimes-confusing world of science and medical technology. We are being asked to evaluate right from wrong in a culture of information sound bites and media-driven arguments.

In his helpful book entitled *Ethics*, Dietrich Bonhoeffer outlined the process by which Christians can strive to make proper, God-pleasing, ethical decisions. First, we must observe and assess the situation and make a decision within the general limitations of human knowledge. Second, we must do what is necessary with a due consideration of reality. Third, our ethical decisions must be bounded by our responsibilities to God and to our neighbors. Fourth, because we live in a sinful world, we might make the wrong decisions even if we honestly think we are doing God's will. Therefore, we completely rely on God's grace for forgiveness if we do the wrong thing whether we know it or not.

So, according to Bonhoeffer, we need to know the facts about an issue before we can even make the proper biblically-informed decision. The purpose of this essay is to present the facts about ESCR in a way that will help Christians better understand what this issue is all about. This will help you take the biblical and confessional principles discussed and appropriately apply them to the controversy over ESCR.

Our bodies have over 100 trillion cells. A cell is the basic building block of life. The largest cells are about the size of a period on a printed page. The smallest ones can only be seen with a microscope. Even though our bodies have so many cells, those cells generate only about 210 different types of tissue cells. We have liver cells, brain cells, muscle cells, kidney cells, bone-producing cells, and so on. All of these cells originally come from one cell called the *zygote*, formed by the union of a male's sperm with a female's egg. The zygote is the very first cell created at conception when a new human being comes into existence. The zygote may also correctly be referred to as an *embryo*. An unborn human being is called an embryo from day 1 to day 60. From day 60 to birth, the baby is termed a *fetus*.

From the moment of its existence, the zygote contains all the instructions necessary to allow it to divide and multiply; however, the zygote doesn't just copy itself. Although the DNA of each cell is the same, certain portions of each cell's genetic information are switched on or off, allowing the cell to *differentiate* (or to change slightly), so each of the 210 different kinds of tissue cells can be produced. This process is not yet fully understood by scientists. These early cells are called *stem cells* because they remind us of the stem of a plant from which grow branches, leaves, and fruit. In a similar way, our body's stem cells are responsible for the 210 types of tissue cells found in our bodies.

Probably the most important point I can make in this essay is that there are two different types of stem cells: *adult* and *embryonic*. *Adult stem cells* are found in your body right now. For example, stem cells found inside our bone marrow produce all the different types of bloods cells we have. Stem cells found in our skin help to restore the many types of skin cells we might lose through injury, disease, or the aging process. Along with our skin and bone marrow, adult stem cells have been discovered in the human heart and brain. Adult stem cells can also be harvested from umbilical cords of newly-born babies and from menstrual blood. You'll see why this is so important in a minute.

Embryonic stem cells, on the other hand, are not found in the bodies of born persons—they can only be taken from embryos. First, researchers use so-called "unwanted" frozen human embryos left over from fertility treatments such as *in vitro fertilization*. Couples decide they no longer want to use these embryos for reproductive purposes, so they are asked by fertility clinics if they would be willing to donate the embryos for research. These embryos are thawed and allowed to grow to the five-day-old stage called the blastocyst, which has about 100 cells. A *blastocyst* reminds me of a poorly-made basketball my brother and I used to play with when we were small. The basketball was lopsided, which made it difficult to make an accurate shot. If we were to cut a blastocyst in half, we would see that it is mostly a hollow ball of cells, with a fluid-filled center. But, like the basketball, the blastocyst is not evenly balanced. One part of the wall is thicker, because this heavier side contains a group of cells called the *inner cell mass*. If the blastocyst were allowed to mature, this clump would eventually form the baby. The blastocyst's outside cells form the other tissues needed to support life in the uterus, such as the placenta and water-filled cushions protecting the baby.

To collect embryonic stem cells, researchers remove the inner cell mass from the rest of the blastocyst. They then put those cells into a petri dish and attempt to stimulate them to grow. These cells are then referred to as a *stem cell line* and can continue to grow almost indefinitely if given the right conditions. Tragically, when the blastocyst, or embryo, is taken apart in this way, it dies. That is what troubles many Christians about ESCR. Embryos are destroyed in the process. If you believe a human person begins at conception, as I do, then people are killed to conduct this research!

Interestingly, most medical researchers who study human development for a living clearly point out that, from a scientific point of view, conception is the only logical event at which we can pinpoint the beginning of a new human life. But often researchers and ethicists who support ESCR will claim that human life only begins when the embryo *implants* into the wall of the uterus, about 14 days after conception. Some would assert that a human being only begins when twinning is no longer likely, or when the nervous system begins its formation, or when

41

the baby could reasonably survive outside of the womb, or even at birth. But if you think about this for a minute, all of these other "events" during the life of a baby simply involve a change in location or a change in its physical anatomy. Only at the time of conception does the genetic information, which makes each of us a unique physical entity, come into existence.

Scientists recognize that there is significant opposition to ESCR, so they have tried to harvest embryonic stem cells from other sources like the reproductive tissues of aborted fetuses. It is also thought that cloning (sometimes called *somatic cell nuclear transfer*, or SCNT) might provide a source for embryonic stem cells. They've even thought about creating genetically-altered embryos so that they couldn't live beyond two weeks of age. They rationalize that, since these mutated embryos couldn't survive anyway, we can do with them as we please. These alternative ways of producing embryonic stem cells seem to create more ethical controversies than they settle. They are also very troubling to Christians who believe it is unethical to create life only to destroy it.

You might be wondering by now why some scientists are so adamant about pursuing stem cell research. They hope to use tissues produced by stem cells for drug or products testing. Right now, adequate drug testing must involve animals or human volunteers. Researchers also hope that studying stem cells will help them to more fully understand cancers and genetic diseases. In fact, they already suspect that cancer is caused by stem cells that have begun to grow abnormally. However, their primary hope is that stem cells might be used to treat previously incurable conditions like Parkinson's disease, diabetes, stroke, heart disease, spinal cord injuries, and arthritis. Politicians, drug companies, universities, and researchers promise "the sky is the limit" where stem cell research is concerned. That brings us to another reason why there is a big push for ESCR. We can't ignore the fact that scientists realize a lot of money, power, and fame is in store for successful embryonic stem cell researchers.

What can we take away from this essay? First, remember that there are two types of stem cells. Adult cells are found in our bodies at this very moment. Their use for treatment should not bother us any more than any other medical treatment, and Christians can wholeheartedly support this type of research in the hope of finding cures. However, research and treatments involving embryonic stem cells are troubling, because human life is sacrificed for the sake of others.

Researchers often argue that the loss of a few zygotes (which they don't believe are human beings) is worth the potential for treating incurable diseases. As of the writing of this essay, no one has been successfully treated with embryonic stem cells. They have caused tissue rejection problems and cancers in lab animals. Many researchers admit that it will be at least 20 years before ESCR will yield any useful treatments, if it ever does. In contrast, right now in excess of 70 treatments are already in use involving *adult* stem cells.

Now that we are aware of the facts surrounding ESCR, we can apply principles from Holy Scripture and the Lutheran Confessions to this issue, as they give us solid biblical guidance for upholding the value of life—from its very beginning.

Embryonic Children and the Value of Life

James Lamb

How small is too small? We can readily answer that question when trying on a pair of jeans! We cannot, however, when it comes to the beginning of life. Dr. Voss states in his essay that, "from a scientific point of view, conception is the only logical event at which we can pinpoint the beginning of a new human life." Science, not size, tells us when life begins. And we can look to Scripture, not size, to tell us when someone is a "child."

Who Is a "Child"?

57. Read Matthew 18:1–5. Who do you suppose the disciples had in mind when they asked, "Who is the greatest?"

58. Jesus turns their focus from themselves to a child. Before addressing their question about the greatest in the Kingdom, He talks about getting into the Kingdom. What two things must they do to enter the kingdom of heaven (v. 3)?

Discuss what it might mean to "become like children" in terms of how we often view children today.

The world of Jesus' day, however, did not always view children the same way we do today. They were not seen as examples of innocence and virtue. Look up Ecclesiastes 10:16; Isaiah 3:4; Isaiah 10:19; 1 Corinthians 3:1; and 1 Corinthians 13:11 and discuss the view of children implied in each.

"In Matthew's Gospel, as in the rest of the Bible, to be 'like a child' is to be weak, in need of protection, unlearned, unable to

44

fend for yourself, small, vulnerable—even when the child is the Son of God (Matthew 2)!"[14]

Based on this biblical understanding, discuss again what it means to "become like children" in order to get into the kingdom of heaven. (See also Matthew 5:3; Romans 3:23; and Philippians 2:5–7.)

Jesus' "backwards" way of doing things recognizes the spiritually helpless as the greatest. They must depend upon Him for life and salvation. This spiritual understanding of ourselves as "children" radically changes the way we view and treat one another. The weakest member of our congregation becomes a "child," and therefore the greatest (see 1 Corinthians 12:20–26)! A "child" is anyone vulnerable and in need (see Matthew 25:34–40).

In light of all the above, discuss this quote by Lutheran ethicist Dr. Gilbert Meilaender: "The embryo is, I believe, the weakest and least advantaged of our fellow human beings, and no community is 'really strong if it will not carry its . . . weakest members' (Karl Barth)."[15]

Prohibitions and Promises about a "Child"

Since the human embryo is by definition human from the moment of conception, and since he or she is completely in need of others for protection and care, it necessarily follows that the human embryo is a human being, a "child" that we are to love and care for. Therefore, what Scripture says about our fellow human beings applies to embryos.

59. Read Exodus 20:13. Does size have anything to do with what constitutes murder? What are the criteria?

---

[14] (Dr. Jeffery Gibbs. *Cherish the Children: Jesus' Backwards Understanding of "Who Is the Greatest."* A Life Sunday Bible study available from Lutherans for Life, Nevada, IA.)
[15] Gilbert Meilaender, "Some Protestant Reflections," *The Human Embryonic Stem Cell Debate: Science, Ethics, and Public Policy*, edited by Suzanne Holland, Karen Lebacqz, and Laurie Zoloth (MIT Press, 2000), 141.

Of course, as Luther reminds us, there is a positive side to this commandment. Read (or recite!) Luther's explanation to the Fifth Commandment. Discuss how this applies to embryos.

Read Exodus 20:3. The First Commandment obviously speaks of our relationship to God. But it also relates to embryonic stem cell research and the embryo. Discuss that relationship based on the following passages: Genesis 11:1–9; Proverbs 3:5–8; Proverbs 14:12; and Matthew 25:37–46.

60. Read Luther's explanation of the First Article of the Apostles' Creed. When did God's provision for all we need for this "body and life" begin? (See Psalm 139:13–14.) How does this relate to embryos in a petri dish or frozen in storage?

But embryonic stem cell research is not just a First Article question.

61. Read Luther's explanation of the Second Article of the Apostles' Creed. How could the phrase, "that I may be His own," be applied to embryos?

Discuss the promises in Romans 6:10; Hebrews 7:27; and 2 Timothy 2:4 and how they relate to the embryo.

Conclusion

Every human being, no matter how small, is someone created by God for whom Jesus Christ died. Every human being, no matter how small, is a "child"—someone vulnerable and in need of our care. What God says in His Word about human beings applies to tiny human embryos. That God Himself became an embryo gives inestimable value to every human embryo.

Lesson 6

Defining Terms: The Importance of Vocabulary in Pursuing Ethics

Maggie Karner

One of the most important things I learned from my former career in healthcare marketing is that proper use of language is critical. It forms the foundation for all our communication and, at least in health professions, often provides for the proper administration of life-saving treatment. Language truly is a matter of life and death.

Language can be used as a creative vehicle and used to carry a message that you want understood or perceived. In this way, language can provide clarity to an issue, or it can be used as "noise" to obscure the real truth of the matter.

Anyone who has studied a foreign tongue understands the limitations of the English language. It is generally understood that the English vocabulary has a limited ability to communicate the hidden nuances of meaning. So I find it comforting that God chose the precise languages of Hebrew and Greek to communicate His *Logos*, or Word, to us. Both these languages are revered for their ability to communicate clearly and to refine subtle meanings in an intentional way. Because of this, God's Word is keen and sharp in the way it presents God's value of human life.

In the Bible, we find unambiguous references to God's passionate love for all human life at every stage of development. We also read about God's prohibition on the taking of human life—even if our feeble motives appear compassionate. In Psalm 139, God specifically says "You knitted me together in my mother's womb. I praise You, for I am fearfully and wonderfully made. . . . My frame was not hidden from You, when I was being made in secret." Even here, our English fails us, because the Hebrew word for *womb* does not only refer to a woman's uterus. Instead, the word refers to all the "inner parts" of a woman where a child is created.

What the Christian can understand from Psalm 139 is that God is busy creating every new "person" from the moment of conception—even while that tiny new human is traveling through the mother's fallopian tube on its way to the uterus.

This semantic detail becomes important today, when many in the scientific community would prefer the public to think that a young embryo is not a "person" until it is implanted in a woman's uterus, less than one week after conception. By stressing personhood upon *implantation*, this also effectively redefines the meaning of the word *pregnant* to mean only when the fertilized embryo attaches to the uterus. This deliberately manipulates the language in an attempt to confuse scientific facts. Most embryology textbooks testify that human life begins at conception—not implantation.

This ploy is used to build acceptance for embryonic stem cell research, genetic testing, pre-genetic diagnosis testing (PGD), and certain birth control products that act as abortifacients. If a tiny one-celled embryo is not perceived as a person, many research scientists hope to garner the support they need to control—and dispose of—thousands of embryos at will, constrained only by their utilitarian, humanist motives.

This is especially true when it comes to embryonic stem cell research and cloning. Despite the mantra that claims embryonic stem cell research only uses "leftover" embryos, researchers know that thousands of additional fresh embryos will be needed to establish enough cell lines for advanced research. Therefore, cloning to produce these embryos for research is inevitable. And every biotech public relations executive knows that the public broadly rejects this research when they understand it involves human cloning. According to an ABC news poll, nearly nine out of ten Americans surveyed believe that human cloning should be illegal.[16]

So how do those in favor of this research get public and private support? It appears that they have simply chosen to obscure the truth of the matter by changing the way in which the matter is discussed and promoted. By changing the language, people can dramatically influence people's opinions.

Pro-cloning researchers often attempt to soften the harsh realities of their agenda by manipulating the language through the use of misleading adjectives. For instance, the popular term *therapeutic cloning* is often used to refer to cloning that creates embryos that are later to be destroyed in embryonic stem cell research. On the other hand, researchers stay away from the term *reproductive cloning*, which is a term they prefer to use when referring to the process for making babies that will be born. They are very aware that this controversial term strikes understandable fear in the hearts of many ethically conscious people. Apparently, proponents of this terminology believe that the end justifies the means, and that destruction of one innocent human life can be deemed "therapy" if it proposes to help somebody else. But simply adding an adjective to the term *cloning* doesn't alter the procedure. The plain truth is that cloning *is* cloning. Sometimes, though, proponents of cloning simply change the definition of the word, deciding that cloning to provide human embryos for research isn't cloning after all.

In 2006, for example, a craftily-worded state constitutional amendment in Missouri to encourage publicly-funded embryonic stem cell research and cloning for this purpose was added as a state ballot referendum. However, the referendum's language was deceptive in that it claimed to "ban cloning." Many voters may not have noticed that, deep in the language of the referendum, the term *cloning* was conveniently redefined. Claiming to seek permission only to allow somatic cell nuclear transfer (or SCNT), the amendment insulted informed Missourians who

---

[16] "Majority Opposes Human Cloning Similar Response to Animal and Therapeutic Uses," ABC News Poll Vault, 3/7/07, <http://abcnews.go.com/sections/scitech/DailyNews/poll010816_cloning.html> This *ABCNEWS*/Beliefnet poll was conducted by telephone August 8–12, 2001, among a random national sample of 1,024 adults. The results have a three-point margin of error. Fieldwork by TNS Intersearch of Horsham, Pa.

knew that SCNT is simply the correct scientific definition of cloning—the same process used to clone Dolly the sheep. The biological fact is that SCNT creates a new human life, a completely distinct human organism. By using scientifically inaccurate language, proponents of this measure essentially hijacked public debate. When the election dust had settled, proponents of the measure had spent nearly $28 million in private funds (most of it from one donor source) attempting to persuade voters that cloning *isn't* cloning. Unfortunately, money *can* buy the language of publicity and the measure passed by a narrow margin.

Christians know all too well that language can be a double-edged sword. Satan has always used language as a tool to deceive us. "Now the serpent was more crafty than any other beast of the field that the Lord God had made. He said to the woman, "Did God actually say, 'You shall not eat of *any* tree in the garden'?" (Genesis 3:1, emphasis mine). And Eve was deceived by Satan's word games. The truth was that God gave Adam and Eve the freedom to eat from *all other trees* of the garden, with the *only exception* being the tree of the knowledge of good and evil.

As a former marketer, I have the greatest respect for the devil's persuasive professionalism. Satan is the world's best marketing executive. He has total command of the language and uses it at his disposal, subtly changing the language of truth into a deception.

But God's Word is unchangeable truth. We know that God's Word is more powerful than any of the tools Satan has as he wishes. "For the word of God is living and active, sharper than any two-edged sword . . . discerning the thoughts and intentions of the heart" (Hebrews 4:12). Armed with that truth, we are prepared to do battle against the deceptive schemes of Satan and his message of death.

We know that God is the author and designer of life, from beginning to end. And we don't have permission to edit His will by "editing" our use of language to support our own human agendas.

Right Words and the Value of Life

James Lamb

Words are important. We use words to describe reality. Unfortunately, some use words to distort reality. Many attempt to distort the reality of life at its very beginnings in order to make something evil appear to be good. Christians, however, have a "reality check"—the truth of God's Word.

"Did God Actually Say?"

Read Genesis 3:1–7. Distorting the truth is nothing new! Note Jesus' comments about this "serpent of old" in John 8:44.

The devil is a liar, but a "crafty" one. A successful counterfeiter of twenty-dollar bills makes the "lie" look as much like the truth as possible. Discuss 2 Corinthians 11:14 and 2 Thessalonians 2:9 with this in mind.

62. What purpose do his lies serve? (See Isaiah 5:20 and Revelation 12:9, 17.)

Compare the serpent's quote of what God said to what God actually said (Genesis 2:16).

The devil does not deny that "God said." He deceives to cast doubt on what God *meant*. From the beginning, the devil would have God's Word be subservient to humanity rather than the other way around. He would have the Word be used according to human whims and desires rather than have it be received as God's revealed truth that makes us "wise for salvation." He distorts the Word of truth, making people think they are the masters of its meaning. When that happens, God's Word is rendered meaningless.

What God Actually Says!

The truth of science speaks to many of the deceptive words used to justify the destruction of human life. People have said, "I'm opposed to cloning, but I am in favor of somatic cell nuclear transfer (SCNT) for the purpose of curing disease." This is a scientific absurdity! It is saying, "I'm opposed to cloning, but I'm in favor of cloning" (see Lesson 6 essay).

63. The truth of God's Word speaks to Christians who try to distort His Word to their liking or buy into the distortions made by society. The following are some examples:

"Right to Choose"

Christians sometimes equate the "right to choose" with Christian freedom. Apply the truth of Deuteronomy 30:11–20; 1 Corinthians 10:23–24; Galatians 5:13; and 1 Peter 2:16 to this distortion.

"Pregnant"

64. Christians can be deceived by the redefinition of *pregnant* to mean implantation in a uterus—as if there is some distinction between human embryos that are implanted and those that are not. What common phrase is found in the following passages? How does it speak to God's view of pregnancy? See Genesis 4:1; 21:2; 29:32; Exodus 2:2; Isaiah 8:3; and Luke 1:31. Also, review what the essay says about the scriptural word for *womb*.

Personhood

The essay mentions that the word *person* gets used to distract us from the central question. The important question is not, "When does personhood begin?" but rather, "When does human life begin?" The answer to the latter is an objective fact of science—conception. The answer to the former is a subjective and philosophical question. God's directives regarding how we treat human life come into play at conception regardless of someone's opinion as to when each of us becomes a person.

Nevertheless, Scripture speaks of unborn human life in a personal way. Discuss this in relation to the following passages: Job 3:3; Psalm 139:13–16; Jeremiah 1:5; and Luke 1:41–44.

"My Body, My Choice"

Biology certainly speaks to the incorrect phrase, "my body, my choice." There are two bodies involved in a pregnancy: the mother's and the baby's. But God's Word also speaks to this in a much more profound way. Discuss this after reading 1 Corinthians 6:19–20.

Fetus versus Baby

Fetus versus *baby* is another word game people play. *Fetus* is a correct biological term for the unborn from eight weeks to birth. But people generally speak of having a "baby." Those sweatshirts with the little arrow say, "Baby on Board"! But people do not like to say, "Baby aborted." So, *fetus* is religiously used by pro-abortion people to dehumanize the baby, trying to make a distinction between born and unborn. But the Bible makes no such distinction.

The Greek word for a very young child is *brephos*. All of the following passages use this word. Discuss the implications this has for the *fetus* versus *baby* word game. See Luke 1:41, 44; Luke 2:12, 16; Luke 18:15; Acts 7:19; 2 Timothy 3:15; and 1 Peter 2:2.

The Hebrew word for "son," used also for "children," is *ben*. Contrast the use of this word in Genesis 17:25 and 25:22.

Conclusion

Words are important, but they can be used to distort reality. Thank God for His Word—His "reality check"!

Lesson 7

Vocation:
Serving God by Serving Our
Neighbor—For Life

Uwe Siemon-Netto

Martin Luther tells us that all of God's children are "priests." We are members of the universal priesthood of all believers. In fact, in this priesthood we render the highest service to God—not in Sunday worship but in the performance of our daily chores. But there's a proviso: Whatever our calling (or "vocation") might be—mother, doctor, scientist, plumber, soldier, policeman, waitress, computer programmer, or President of the United States—we must exercise it to the best of our abilities out of love for our neighbor.

Then, and only then, says Luther, are we God's agents, God's partners, God's cooperators. Luther explained that we are "masks" behind which God hides and through which He acts in His secular realm.

Years ago in a Chicago seminary, a female divinity student protested: "But God never asked *me* if I wished to be called to bear a child." Well, yes, that's true. He didn't. God does not *force* us to be His mask as mother or father. He does not *force* us to be His mask in any vocation. But here we must remember that if we are not God's mask, we are none other than the devil's mask. There is no in-between.

So we function as God's masks when we work well in our vocations for our neighbors' benefit. This is not to say that we must not reap profit from our labor; nowhere does the Bible say that we should not make money from our calling, if indeed our calling is a moneymaking enterprise (such as our job). After all, it is certainly a noble vocation to feed our families and ourselves.

Where things go wrong is when we make ourselves the main focus of our work. When we pander to the contemporary "me" culture, then we cease to be God's mask. Instead, we become a mask of His adversary, the devil. In our secular vocations, a Christian's eye must be firmly on the you—on the neighbor. Serving him or her means serving God.

I won't delve into the many callings of growing and adult persons going through life from the crèche to the grave. I believe my message is clear: our *Gottesdienst*, our service to God, is not limited to Sunday worship and prayers before meals. We serve Him by serving others in all our worldly functions—no, not by evangelizing our colleagues as they are busy writing a complicated computer program or exercising their own vocations, but just by doing our own work out of love for others—our neighbors.

But who is our neighbor? Christ makes this very clear in Matthew 25: the naked, the thirsty, the hungry, the sick, and the poor. As He said, "Truly, I say to you, as you did it to one of the least of these My brothers, you did it to Me" (Matthew 25:40). The list can be continued at will. It includes the client, the boss, the subordinate, the guy behind the wheel of the other car on the way to work. In fact, anybody created by God is our neighbor.

Let's start then with the smallest and most defenseless neighbor—the human embryo—a complete person at whose very conception all the DNA information transferred from the father to the mother's egg would fill thousands of volumes in a library. So how do we serve that little embryo—or for that matter, the millions of other unborn babies in the womb at various stages of development? By loving the baby in advance of his or her birth. By making the mother's womb the closest approximation of paradise—a secure and healthy location. By working to enact just and moral laws that protect the right of each child to remain safe in the womb. By not exposing the child to external dangers and, presumably, to dangers of the soul. By letting the sounds of wonderful music penetrate this parapet of the warm paradise in which the child temporary resides. By praying for safe delivery. Then, by caring for the mother and the young family as they face the challenges of modern life. That's it. If we do that, we serve God. We are His disguise, His mask, His partner.

Let's remain with the smallest humans: if the child is already a person created by God, is he or she also God's mask? Do embryos and other unborn children have a calling? I submit that they do—if only because they *are* persons. But what might that calling be? Well, for one thing, they are called to receive love and respect from others, a vocation that also applies to a dying person. We can think of this as a "passive" vocation. Those in service to them receive great benefit from this relationship of "server" to "the served." The closest analogy is the function of a pastor quietly hearing confession, or of a psychiatrist listening to his patient.

Unborn children are called to receive love inside the womb, love from their parents. However, they are presumably also called to prepare themselves to give love to their parents once they are born. The most striking evidence for this is the pure and unfailing love given by children with Down syndrome. Due to prenatal testing, these children have become a rarity, because babies suspected to have Down syndrome are almost routinely aborted these days. This is a tragedy not just for these very real persons—and against God—but also for their parents, who will never know the joy of receiving overwhelming love from such wonderful kids.

In the universal priesthood of all believers, it is our worldly calling to enable our younger and defenseless neighbors to exercise their vocation upon us—their older, and more developed, neighbors. In other words, just like the defenseless baby in her mother's womb, the endangered embryo has the passive calling to enable caring Christians to be priests in the secular realm as we work to show the value of her life.

"Being Neighbor" and the Value of Life

James Lamb

Everyone knows Mr. Rogers's melodious question, "Would you be mine? Could you be mine? Won't you be my neighbor?" If we listen closely to the tiniest of human beings—embryos in fallopian tubes and wombs, embryos in petri dishes and fertility clinic storage—we might also hear, "Won't you be my neighbor?" If we listen closely to God's Word, we will hear Him saying, "I have been 'neighbor' to you in Jesus. Be 'neighbor' to others."

The Importance of "Being Neighbor"

65. Read Mark 12:29–31. According to Jesus, what is the second greatest thing a person could possibly do? Relate this to the greatest thing a person could possibly do.

66. How do Romans 13:8–10 and Galatians 5:14 give importance to loving our neighbor?

67. Review the Fourth through Tenth Commandments (Exodus 20:12–17). Briefly discuss each in terms of our daily relationship with our neighbor through the vocation (see Lesson 7) to which God calls us. Focus on what we are not to do.

The Purpose of "Being Neighbor"

68. What do Romans 15:2; 1 Corinthians 10:24; and Galatians 6:2 say about the purpose of "being neighbor" through our vocations?

Using the explanation of the Fourth through Tenth Commandments in Luther's Small Catechism, discuss each commandment, focusing on what we are to do as we relate to our neighbor through our vocations.

Who Is My Neighbor?

We assume correctly in the above discussions that our neighbor is anyone with whom we have contact in our vocations. But Scripture sometimes narrows that focus.

69. Read Luke 10:25–37. This most famous "neighbor" story in the Bible starts as a "salvation" story: "What shall I do to inherit eternal life?" (v. 25) To what does Jesus point this self-righteous lawyer?

70. The lawyer comes up with the correct answer according to the Law (Deuteronomy 6:5 and Leviticus 19:18). What do you suppose is behind the famous "Who is my neighbor?" question?

71. Discuss how people today seek to justify themselves by limiting who they see as their neighbor. How might this relate to embryonic stem cell research or abortion?

72. Jesus turns the tables a bit and frames "neighbor" as the doer, not recipient, of the action. "Which of these three, do you think, proved to be a neighbor to the man who fell among the robbers?" (Luke 10:36). Based on what it means to be neighborly, "The one who showed him mercy" (v. 37), who then is especially our neighbor?

Relate this to Matthew 18:5; Matthew 25:34–40; and James 1:27.

The phrases "one such child," "least of these," and "orphans and widows" describe neighbors especially in need of love and mercy. Discuss how these phrases apply to human embryos and babies not yet born. Discuss how they apply to the frail elderly or those with severe disabilities.

73. We do not always have contact with these most vulnerable neighbors. Nevertheless, how can we "be neighbor" to them in our daily vocations? (See Proverbs 31:8–9 and Psalm 82:3–4.)

Discuss this also in light of the quote from Dr. Siemon-Netto's essay, "We are 'masks' behind which God hides and through which He acts in His secular realm."

A pastor tells his homebound members and those in care centers, "By allowing me to serve you, you are Jesus to me. Thank you!" (See again Matthew 25:40.) Discuss in what sense being the recipients of love can be a vocation.

God "Being Neighbor"

Like the lawyer in the Good Samaritan story, we live under the Law if we think the job will be accomplished just by telling ourselves or others, "Love your neighbor!"

74. Read Ephesians 2:1–3. By nature, how neighborly are we?

75. Read Ephesians 4:4–10. "But God" is neighborly! He loved us with a "great love." Where do we see our "neighborliness" in these verses? Where does it come from?

76. Where does service to neighbor come from? (See Mark 10:45 and John 13:12–14.)

77. Where does love for neighbor come from? (See 1 John 4:7–11.)

78. Where does our vocation come from? When do we get it? (See Psalm 139:16.)

This is a good place to remind ourselves of the neighbors among us (maybe even us) hurting because of mistakes against our tiniest neighbors—a past abortion or struggles over reproductive technology decisions. God loves these neighbors and speaks clearly to them (and us). (See 1 John 1:5–9.)

Discuss this statement: "Being neighbor flows from what God has done and still does for us and through us!"

Conclusion

God said, "Yes" to us! We can say "Yes!" to those we deal with in our vocations and joyfully defend and speak up for the least and most vulnerable in our society.

Lesson 8

God's Two Kingdoms: Honoring Life's Value in Our World

Charles P. Arand

Christians in the twenty-first century live in an uncharted, post-modern world. That world no longer shares the moral foundations of a western society shaped by Christianity for seventeen hundred years. In such a new era, how shall Christians work together with non-Christians to make responsible decisions in the area of civil legislation, public policy, social programs, and bioethics? How can we actively honor the sanctity of life in our world? In order to navigate the complexities of our day, Lutherans need to draw upon and develop an underutilized resource known as the distinction between the two kingdoms or God's two forms of governance.

Two Hands—Two Forms of Governance

Although the phrase *doctrine of two kingdoms* is of relatively recent origin, the concept of two kingdoms traces its roots back to the New Testament.[17] Martin Luther used the language of two kingdoms in several ways.[18] He used it most often to distinguish

---

[17] Matthew 22:14–22; Rom 13:1ff; Rom 2:11. For a historical overview of the concept within the Christian tradition, see Karl H. Hertz, ed., *Two Kingdoms and One World: A Sourcebook in Christian Ethics* (Minneapolis: Augsburg Publishing House, 1976).

[18] For example, he could also use it to refer to the kingdom of God versus the kingdom of Satan and such. For an overview of this distinction and concept, see Robert Kolb, "Two Kingdoms Doctrine," in *The Encyclopedia of Christianity*, vol. 3. Edited by Erwin Fahlbusch, et al., (Grand Rapids, Eerdmans; Leiden, Brill, 1999–2005). For further reading, see Robert

God's activity within the vertical (our life with God) and horizontal (our life with one another) dimensions of human life. Luther labeled the vertical dimension of life the "right-hand," "spiritual," or "heavenly" realm. He labeled the horizontal dimension of life the "left-hand," "temporal," or "earthly" realm.

With His right hand, God gathers to Himself from the four corners of the world a community of believers known as the one holy Christian Church. In the death and resurrection of His Son, God reestablishes communion with His human creatures. Through the Gospel in its various forms, God sends the Spirit of His Son to impart new birth to eternal life. In this way, God creates, governs, preserves, strengthens, and sustains a community of believers who share the same Jesus Christ and Holy Spirit in the midst of a sin-wracked world. But this realm is visible only to God. Only Christians experience life under the right hand of God.

With His left hand, God preserves and protects human life in our relationships with one another. God has placed every human being into various walks of life, including family and economic life, political and social life, and the Church or religious life.[19] Within these arenas, human beings exercise certain responsibilities and tasks (that Christians perceive as callings) that are regulated by God's Law. Both believers and unbelievers experience life under the left hand of God. Working through human beings in these offices as His "masks," God uses just laws and government, civic-minded workers, and everyday occupations to preserve the human community from complete destruction under the onslaught of sin. Through this left-hand

---

Benne, *The Paradoxical Vision: A Public Theology for the Twenty-first Century* (Minneapolis: Augsburg, 1995) and Uwe Siemon-Netto, *The Fabricated Luther. The Rise and Fall of the Shirer Myth* (St. Louis: Concordia Publishing House, 1995).

[19] In the right-hand realm of God, the Church is considered in its nature as an assembly or gathering of believers. In the left-hand realm of God we can also consider the Church as an institution in as much as it is constituted by a constitution, governed by by-laws, obeys zoning laws, and such. When Americans think of the separation of church and state it has to do with the distinction between the church as an institution and the government as an institution. Both reside in what Luther would call the left-hand realm. Thus, the American separation of church and state is not identical with Luther's distinction of the two realms.

realm, God protects society from disorder and chaos—which, in turn, enables the Church (or right-hand realm) to more effectively proclaim the saving news of the Gospel.

Although Christians live in both realms simultaneously, our interest here concerns how Christians work within God's left hand in the horizontal realm. During the course of American history, Lutherans have raised families and contributed to the economy through their labor. They have established educational and charitable institutions in order to attend to the temporal needs of others within society. But when it comes to political matters and the larger social issues that have political implications, Lutherans of German descent have been nearly invisible and their voice unheard by the larger Christian and non-Christian community.

Historical factors may have contributed to the lack of Lutheran influence in political affairs. Luther held deep fears of disorder and chaos, shaped by peasant revolts, and so desired a strong government. This remained the case for Lutherans in Germany throughout the nineteenth century. Thus, when German Lutherans immigrated to America, they came from a non-democratic society in which peasants did not actively participate. Their role in relation to the state and institutional Church could be described as "pray, pay, and obey."

Theologically, Lutherans have at times focused on the ultimate importance of salvation and eternal life in such a way that it had the unintended effect of disparaging life in a world that is passing away. Some would propose that as we await the world to come, "we place our rears as comfortably as we can into our secular reality, leaving it to others to dirty their hands in political filth" (Siemon-Netto). Some would argue that such a view led to quietistic indifference among Lutherans and subservience to secular authority. Both views misunderstand Luther's distinction of the two realms. God calls Christians to be human—and active—in both realms.

Characteristics of Life in God's Left Hand

In the Creed, Lutherans affirm the goodness of the world when we confess that God created the world and continues to govern it. We reaffirm its value when we confess that Christ died for the world. And so Christians respond to the fallen world (even as Christ did) not by flight into Christian colonies but "by standing tall, rolling up one's sleeves, and saying, 'I am not going anywhere; this world has been bought by Christ and his [work], and I am going to serve by living life as he intended it to be.'"[20] The reformers of the sixteenth century reclaimed the sphere of secular government as a legitimate and proper scope for Christian living and vocational service—in contrast to the monastic life, so common in that day, in which people retreated from the world.

In His left-hand realm, God works through creatures as His masks behind which He acts as the creative agent of life. Luther describes creatures as "the hands, channels, and means through which God bestows all blessings. For example, he gives to the mother breasts and milk for her infant, and he gives grain and all kinds of fruits from the earth for man's nourishment—things which no creature could produce by himself."[21] Even after the fall into sin, parents, farmers, carpenters, employers, and doctors continue to function as God's instruments for the well-being of society, even if they do so unwittingly. Christians see that through the needs of our neighbor God calls us to live as His co-workers for the temporal and physical well-being of others.

The responsibilities and tasks of our formal roles as parents, workers, and citizens are given substance and form by the Law that God wove into the very fabric of creation itself—known as "natural law" or the "law of creation." In a sense, it describes the grain of the universe. As such, it provides common ground for social action in cooperation with non-Christians. The violation of these norms results in the undoing of human community. For example, marriages fall apart when spouses demean and abuse one another. Divorce divides families. Homosexuality is not the social equivalent of heterosexuality. The stability of a community is undermined when people rob and harm one another. And in today's society, complicated ethical issues in science, research, and medicine threaten to undo the moral fabric of our human community.

---

[20] Robert Rosin, "Christians and Culture: Finding Place in Clio's Mansions," *Christ and Culture: The Church in a Post-Christian(?) America* (St. Louis: Concordia Seminary Monograph Series, 1995), 69.
[21] Large Catechism I, 26. *The Book of Concord: The Confessions of the Evangelical Lutheran Church* (Philadelphia: Fortress Press, 2000).

Although Luther rejected any contribution of reason to our justification before God ("I cannot by my own reason or strength believe in Jesus Christ my Lord."), he extols reason as a gift of God in creation ("He has given me reason and all my senses."). In particular, God has given human beings brains so that they might work to create just and moral laws to serve the various needs of life. Here Luther values the reasoning abilities of non-Christians as well as Christians. And so it is rumored that he quipped, "it is better to have a wise Turk than a foolish Christian as a ruler." The point here is that Christians cannot claim special insight into public policy or social programs based on the Gospel. Likewise, the freedom and wisdom of the Gospel is lost on the secular world. It can only apply to those who understand God's saving grace—those living in His right-hand realm. However, Christians are free to utilize insights from disciplines such as political theory, social ethics, bioethics, and family therapy in determining how best to serve the neighbor in the kingdom of God's left hand.

As we look after the bodily well-being of our neighbor, human imagination identifies various possibilities for dealing with social issues. We can recognize that there is not always a "right" way or "wrong" solution. Instead, patient, reasoned debate determines better and worse ways to serve the neighbor. Christians may agree that everyone should have access to health care but are free to disagree on how we can best achieve it. Furthermore, we must realize that today's "better" way may look worse tomorrow.[22]

Finally, Luther's distinction of the two realms recognizes that, this side of eternity, we will never find the "perfect solution" to the social problems of our day, much less establish a utopia on earth. Human activity in creation cannot and does not eliminate sin. That belongs to the work of Christ. Working with God's left hand, human activity serves to stem the tide of evil and hold things together until Christ returns—and to provide free and fertile ground for the work of the right-hand kingdom in proclaiming the Gospel. This is why it is critical for Christians to

---

[22] Mary Jane Haemig, "The Confessional Basis of Lutheran Thinking on Church-State Issues," *Church and State: Lutheran Perspectives*, ed. John R. Stumme and Robert W. Tuttle (Philadelphia: Fortress Press, 2003), 14.

value the opportunity to engage in the public policy discussions of the left-hand realm. By educating and informing our reason, Christians can influence the debate, work to create just laws and ethical boundaries, and provide protection for society's most vulnerable members.

Conclusion

"He's got the whole world in His hands." The entire world belongs to God. But as He holds the entire world in both hands, God deals with His human creatures in two different ways. He creates and preserves the Church through the Gospel. He regulates human affairs through the Law. As Christians, we are called to live in our vertical relationship with God by faith and in horizontal relationships responsibly with one another by love, even if that means getting our hands "dirty" in the secular world of life.

Lights in a Dark World and the Value of Life

James Lamb

From its beginning, Christianity influenced the world. Christians "turned the world upside down" (Acts 17:6) through the power of the Gospel proclaimed (Mark 16:15) and lived (James 1:22–26). From adopting babies exposed by the Romans to providing care for the dying, Christians brought light into a dark world.

The need for Christian influence on society remains vital, especially when it comes to assaults on the very beginnings of life. But aren't things like abortion and embryonic stem cell research political issues? Should Christians be involved in political issues or are we just called to proclaim the Gospel? The answer is, "Yes!"

The Light of the World

Jesus is the light of the world. Discuss the need for the Light and the hope of the Light. See Isaiah 60:1–3; John 3:16–21; John 8:12; and John 12:46.

The Lights in the World

79. Read Colossians 1:11–14 and 1 Peter 2:9. The Light of the world calls us into His kingdom as lights!

How does this relate to Mark 15:33 and 2 Corinthians 5:21?

The Light of the world works through His lights in the world. Read Matthew 5:14–16.

80. The *you* in verse 14 is plural in the Greek. (See also John 12:36 and Ephesians 5:8.) Why is that encouraging?

81. What is the ultimate purpose of being lights?

Lights and Government

82. Which of the following best reflects a Christian's responsibility toward government according to Matthew 22:15–22: "God or Government" or "God and Government"? Why?

83. How does Jesus' prayer for His apostles in John 17:11, 14–18 speak to all Christians and our relationship to government?

84. Where do governments come from, and why do they exist? (See Romans 13:1–7.)

Think about the kind of government Paul lived under when he wrote Romans 13.

85. Must Paul's admonitions be carried out absolutely? (See Acts 5:29.)

Lights and Life

We have reviewed the focus of Dr. Arand's essay. Christians simultaneously live in God's right-hand kingdom: His rule of grace through the Gospel—and His left-hand kingdom: His rule of law through governments. We are called *by* the Light in the former and *to be* lights in the latter. The call to "be lights" involves more than passively "glowing in the dark"!

86. Read Ephesians 5:8–11. Action words such as *walk* are associated with those who are "light in the Lord." Discuss what it means for children of light to "walk." What is the "fruit of light"? (See Galatians 5:22–23; Philippians 1:11; and Colossians 1:10.)

87. Relate this to Lesson 7 and our "neighborly" vocations. How would our walk produce fruit in the following?
- Holding a position in government
- Discussing a local bond issue
- Voting
- Serving in the military

The purpose of such "walking" is not just to be "nice." Review the purpose (Matthew 5:16).

Take No Part

88. Children of light are to have nothing to do with "unfruitful works of darkness." It becomes imperative, then, to discern such works. How do we define "works of darkness"? (See John 17:17; 2 Corinthians 4:2; and 2 Timothy 3:16.) Which of the following would be "works of darkness"?

• A school bond issue you think will raise property taxes too much
• A Republican plan to save Social Security
• A Democratic plan to save Social Security
• Signing a petition to remove all restrictions on abortion in your state.

Expose

Ephesians 5:11, however, calls for more than avoidance. "Expose" is a strong, direct, action word. When government actions attack God and His truth, His "lights" are compelled to speak and act. Bills to fund embryonic stem cell research or abortion are more than political issues. As we have seen in previous lessons, these intentionally destroy human life. They, therefore, attack the Author and Redeemer of life.

89. In exposing "works of darkness" to fellow Christians, what is our approach? (See Paul's approach in Acts 17:2–3.)

90. What approach can we use in the secular realm? (See Paul's approach in Acts 17:22–34.)

91. Exposing "works of darkness" goes beyond boldly calling wrong things wrong. It becomes an opportunity to help people see the Light. Who does Paul end up proclaiming, both in Thessalonica and Athens?

Conclusion

God calls Christians in His right-hand kingdom and makes them His "lights." He calls them to be involved in the left-hand kingdom by letting their light shine in all they do. He calls them to expose that which assaults Him. He calls them to take advantage of every opportunity to glorify Him by proclaiming Jesus!

Further Resources

For more information about embryonic stem cell research and other medical and scientific issues, see the following.

Books

Holy People, Holy Lives: Law and Gospel in Bioethics, Richard C. Eyer. St. Louis: Concordia Publishing House, 2000.

BioEngagement: Making a Christian Difference Through Bioethics Today, Nigel M. de S. Cameron, Scott E. Daniels, Barbara White, editors. Grand Rapids, Mich.: Wm. B. Eerdmans Publishing Company, 2000.

Consumer's Guide to a Brave New World, Wesley J. Smith. San Francisco: Encounter Books, 2004.

Human Dignity in the Biotech Century: A Christian Vision for Public Policy, Charles W. Colson and Nigel M. de S. Cameron, editors. Downers Grove, Ill.: InterVarsity Press, 2004.

LCMS World Relief and Human Care Resources

Life Ministries
1333 S. Kirkwood Road
St. Louis, MO 63122
(800) 248-1930, ext. 1380
worldrelief.lcms.org

LCMS Life Ministries Notes for Life e-mail newsletter archives

LCMS Life Ministries Online Life Library: "Bioethics" and "Cloning."

A large online collection of papers, articles, and information on life issues. Simply click on one of the topics above for a complete list and summaries of our available information. The information there is online, free of charge, and easily downloaded.

A Small Catechism on Human Life, John T. Pless, LCMS World

Relief and Human Care, 2006.

This is available through Concordia Publishing House, www.cph.org or 1-800-325-3040.

A Small Catechism on Human Life, Simplified for Younger Readers, John T. Pless and Michelle Bauman, LCMS World Relief and Human Care, 2006.

This is available through Concordia Publishing House, www.cph.org or 1-800-325-3040.

Lutherans For Life Resources

Lutherans For Life
1120 South G Avenue
Nevada, IA 50201
www.lutheransforlife.org

God's Word for Life—A comprehensive study Bible containing thirty-eight commentaries or articles connecting the life issues to God's Word.

The 3 Bs of When Life Begins—If the "3Rs" are the basics of education, the "3Bs" are the basics of when life begins—biology, Bible, and Baptism.

Cloning: Understanding the Basics—A simple explanation of the cloning process and how God's Word speaks to this technology.

Emergency Contraception—A look at what "Emergency Contraception" really means.

In Vitro Fertilization: Moral or Immoral?—Dr. Richard C. Eyer attempts to identify the issues and their moral standing so that the reader can evaluate the moral acceptability or unacceptability of *in vitro* fertilization.

Life before Birth—A full color, pocket-sized brochure with beautiful photographs of the pre-born child developing through the first nine months of life.

Marriage: A Statement by Lutherans For Life—It is important to understand the context God gives for His procreative process.

Stem Cell Research: Understanding the Basics—A simple explanation of this research and how God's Word speaks to this technology.

DVD *Stem Cell Research and Cloning 101: A Primer*—Hosted by Rev. Dr. James I. Lamb (37 minutes).

Watch Me Grow—This beautifully illustrated full-color brochure documents the growth stages of a baby for nine months in the womb.

What about the Facts of Life?—Do you know the amazing facts about the first nine months of your life? This excellent full-color brochure will tell you.

DVD *You Are a Masterpiece*—The amazing world of life before birth is revealed in this live-action video.

Concordia Bioethics Institute Resources

Concordia Bioethics Institute (CBI)
Concordia University Wisconsin
12800 North Lake Shore Drive
Mequon, WI 53097-2402
www.concordiabioethics.org

CBI Tentatio newsletter online archives, covering topics for the Church in post-modern times

CBI Update newsletter online archives

Bible Studies

Playing God: Redesigning Life, Faith on the Edge Series, Robert W. Weise (CPH, 2002).

Six Sessions—*Playing God* explores the ethics of "perfecting" humanity through DNA, cloning, stem cell research, and more. Available at www.cph.org or 1-800-325-3040.

Changing Currents: *Embryonic Stem Cell Research*, Robert C. Baker and Robert W. Weise (CPH, 2005).

One Session—*Embryonic Stem Cell Research* looks at what the Bible says about this controversial topic. By focusing on key Scripture passages concerning the blessings of having children, God's work in procreation, and His prohibition

74

against murder, the study clearly affirms that "life begins at conception" and advocates for responsible scientific and medical research that does not destroy human life. Available at www.cph.org or 1-800-325-3040.

Web Resources

LCMS World Relief and Human Care: worldrelief.lcms.org

Lutherans For Life: www.lutheransforlife.org

Concordia Bioethics Institute:
    www.cuw.edu/Academics/institutes/bioethics/index.html

The Center for Bioethics and Culture (CBC): www.cbc-network.org

The President's Council on Bioethics: www.bioethics.gov

Family Research Council: www.frc.org

Discovery Institute: www.discovery.org/bioethics/

The Center for Bioethics & Human Dignity (CBHD):
    www.cbhd.org

The Snowflakes™ Embryo Adoption program:
    www.nightlight.org/snowflakeadoption.htm

Glossary

adult stem cell research (ASCR). Scientific experimentation on adult stem cells derived from blood, bone marrow, fat, and so forth. ASCR also utilizes blood from discarded human umbilical cords and placentas, but does not result in embryonic death in order to obtain stem cells.

artificial insemination. The introduction of semen into the uterus or oviduct by other than natural means.

bioethics. A discipline dealing with the ethical implications of biological research and applications, especially in medicine

blastocyst. An embryo (day 4–5 of development) shaped like a hollow sphere and containing an inner mass of cells (stem cells) that, left alone, will develop into a fetal human being. Ironically, blastocysts are used in in vitro fertilization (IVF) techniques in order to produce pregnancy, and are destroyed in ESCR in order to obtain stem cells for scientific research.

chromosome. Chromosomes are long pieces of DNA. They are microscopic units containing organized genetic information, located in the nuclei of cells (e.g., human somatic and sex cells), and are also present in one-cell organisms like bacteria, which do not have an organized nucleus. The sum-total of genetic information contained in different chromosomes of a given individual or species are generically referred to as the genome. Chromosomes come in pairs. In humans, the nucleus of each cell has 23 pairs of chromosomes (46 total chromosomes). All of your genes are contained within these 46 nuclear chromosomes and 1 mitochondrial chromosome. Two of the chromosomes (the X and the Y chromosome) determine your gender and are called sex chromosomes.

deoxyribonucleic acid (DNA). An organic substance that encodes and carries genetic information and is the fundamental element of heredity.

embryo. According to *Human Embryology and Teratology*, third edition, Ronan O'Rahilly and Fabiola Müller (New York:

Wiley-Liss, 2001), the official textbook on embryology, the stage of human development beginning with fertilization (and the formation of the zygote) and lasting about nine weeks, after which the developing human being is called a fetus. This textbook also equates the human embryo with an unborn human (p. 8).

embryo adoption. When a family has been successful in having a child through in vitro fertilization, remaining embryos are often cryo-preserved. The frozen embryo adoption program has been named Snowflakes, because embryos are unique and fragile, just like a snowflake. This program began in 1997 to allow embryos to achieve their ultimate purpose—life. Currently, there are over 400,000 frozen embryos in cryo-banks in the United States. These are pre-born children waiting for a chance at life.

embryonic stem cell research (ESCR). Scientific experimentation on stem cells derived from human embryos (usually at the blastocyst stage of development). ESCR results in the destruction of human embryos.

ethics. The field of study examining moral principles or values encompassing law, philosophy, and religion, and applied to a variety of other fields including scientific and medical research. Practitioners in this field are called ethicists.

fallopian tube. Either of the pair of tubes that carry the egg from the ovary to the uterus.

fetus. A developing human being from about nine weeks to birth.

gamete. A sex, or reproductive, cell containing half of the genetic material necessary to form a complete organism. During fertilization, male and female gametes fuse, producing a diploid (i.e., containing paired chromosomes) zygote.

gamete intrafallopian transfer (GIFT). Gametes, both eggs and sperm, are collected and placed together into a catheter. They are both placed into the fallopian tube, where fertilization occurs.

implantation. The process of attachment of the early embryo to the maternal uterine wall.

incarnation. The union of divinity with humanity in Jesus Christ; when God became man.

intracytoplasmic sperm injection (ICSI). Sperm and eggs are collected. Using microsurgical techniques, a single sperm is injected into an egg. The fertilized egg is allowed to grow and is placed into the uterus.

in vitro fertilization (IVF). Sperm and eggs are collected and brought together in a special medium in a petri dish. Sperm spontaneously fertilize the eggs, forming zygotes. The zygotes are allowed to divide and are then placed into the uterus, where it is hoped they will implant and continue to grow. With IVF, the sperm and the egg may, or may not be, from a married couple. With in vitro fertilization, several embryos are created, but only a few are implanted, leaving the remaining embryos to be stored until needed or until they die, are destroyed, or are used for research.

oocyte. The scientific term for the female germ or sex cell produced in the ovaries. It is sometimes erroneously referred to as a human "egg."

somatic cell nuclear transfer (SCNT). This technique is currently the basis for cloning animals (such as the famous Dolly the sheep), and in theory could be used to clone humans. Some researchers use SCNT in embryonic stem cell research. The aim of carrying out this procedure is to obtain stem cells that are genetically matched to the donor organism.

uterus. The muscular female organ for containing and nourishing the young during development prior to birth—sometimes also called the womb.

Yahweh. The English translation of the four Hebrew letters usually transliterated YHWH or JHVH that form a biblical proper name of God.

zygote. The one-cell embryo resulting from the genetic union of a sperm and oocyte; the first stage of embryonic human life.

zygote intrafallopian transfer (ZIFT). A method of assisting reproduction in cases of infertility that is similar to gamete intrafallopian transfer but in which eggs are fertilized in vitro and some of the resulting fertilized eggs are inserted into a fallopian tube.

Authors

Rev. Dr. Charles P. Arand holds the Waldemar and June Schuette Chair in Systematic Theology at Concordia Seminary in St. Louis, Missouri. He is the author of several books including, *Testing the Boundaries: Windows into Lutheran Identity* and *That I May Be His Own: An Overview of Luther's Catechisms*.

Rev. Dr. Albert Collver serves as the executive pastoral assistant for LCMS World Relief and Human Care. He has served in the parish, taught at Concordia University, Ann Arbor, Michigan and has authored several articles.

Dr. Debra L. Schaeffer Grime is an OB/GYN working in the Labor and Delivery Department at Missouri Baptist Medical Center in St. Louis, Missouri.

Rev. Matthew Harrison is the Executive Director of the LCMS World Relief and Human Care Department. He has translated several books and articles from German and Latin, served as editor of *The Lonely Way*, authored several articles and pamphlets, and will soon have a book published.

Rev. Dr. Arthur A. Just, Jr. is the Dean of the Chapel, Director of Deaconess Studies, Co-Director of The Good Shepherd Institute, and Professor of Exegetical Theology at Concordia Theological Seminary, Fort Wayne, Indiana. Dr. Just was a member of the Steering Committee of *Lutheran Service Book* and is the author of *The Ongoing Feast*, the Concordia Commentary on *Luke*, and the Lukan volume of the *Ancient Christian Commentary on Scripture,* and an editor of *Visitation: Resources for the Care for the Soul*.

Maggie Karner chairs the LCMS Sanctity of Human Life Committee and serves as Director of Life Ministries, a program of LCMS World Relief and Human Care.

Rev. Dr. James Lamb serves as the Executive Director of Lutherans For Life, a national organization that witnesses to the sanctity of human life through education based on the Word of God.

Dr. Uwe Siemon-Netto, a veteran international journalist, is scholar in residence and director of the Concordia Seminary Institute on Lay Vocation, St. Louis, Missouri and director of the Concordia Center for Faith and Journalism at Concordia College, Bronxville, New York.

Rev. Dr. Kevin Voss is the Director of the Concordia Bioethics Institute and an Assistant Professor of Philosophy at Concordia University, Mequon, Wisconsin. He is a Doctor of Veterinary Medicine and is currently earning his Ph.D. in Health Care Ethics at Saint Louis University.